BODYB FOR TEENS

By Ben Doughty

ABOUT THE AUTHOR-Ben's Journey

Ever since the age of eleven... yes you heard me right, eleven! I have had a passion for weightlifting, fitness and getting stronger. Now at the age of seventeen, I want to help those who have the same questions that I had about starting weightlifting. When I was starting out, I relied on magazines that were too advanced for the beginner as well as videos online that were cons to open your wallet. After the long process of sorting through these sources and learning through what worked and what was a waste of time, I can now present you with a straightforward and refined guide about how to build your body as a teenager. This is a compiled textbook, Bible, manual, resource, of essential information about bodybuilding and weightlifting for young people.

Bodybuilding has been a great mentor to me, as it has proven to me at such an early age that hard work pays off and that the detail and consistency that is needed in training, can be applied in all walks of life.

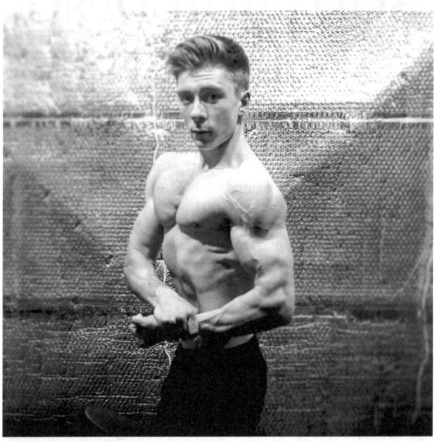

MY STORY

I developed this dream to attain a superhuman physique, after reading bodybuilding magazines in the local barber shop. Inside the magazine was Dorian Yates, this huge mass-monster lifting weights in these grainy, black and white photos. His arms and chest, massive, and legs like tree trunks. I was enthused by the programmes and interviews of the bodybuilders within the magazine. As soon as I was home, I went in search to find my Dad's dumbbells and began doing sets of pushups and situps and shoulder presses. Looking back, it was like I had found my calling, something telling me, "This is it Ben, this is your passion" and every weight that I lifted was the best feeling ever, and seeing the results each week was a huge high.

When I was starting out with this bodybuilding business, I had no equipment apart from a pair of light 4.5KG dumbbells. For the first year I worked on pushups every morning and night, with endless sets of sit ups. These two bodyweight exercises acted as my foundation point to building upper body strength, and they are some of the exercises that I recommend to anyone who is thinking of beginning weight training. They require no equipment, and the secret is... they work! I remember at age twelve reaching pushup numbers into the high seventies for multiple sets and performing hundreds of crunches at a time. From starting out with a maximum of about 10 pushups, I built this number through constant practice, reaching the sweet number of Fifty reps within a few months!

The photo below is of a twelve year old me after a few months of working out with just push-ups, situps and very light dumbbell work. It proves all these online fitness guys wrong, who preach about heavy lifting and costly supplements and expensive gyms. Just hard, consistent work and using the basic equipment and resources around you, can provide you with unlimited results without the need of thousand-pound gym machines.

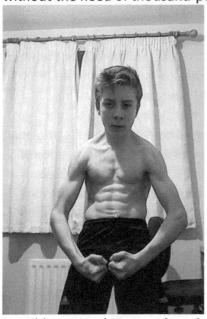

Roughly at age thirteen, I bought a bench press, a small five foot barbell, some weight plates and transformed a one car garage into my gym. These few pieces of basic equipment have stoked my hard training all the way up until this point. Simplicity has always worked and for anyone wanting to begin bodybuilding, the answer is that: all you need is determination and creativity. You can make the same gains as someone training in the skylight-lit, high-tech gym, with only a few dusty weights and a vivid dream. The garage would reach scorching temperatures of thirty-plus degrees in the summer and below freezing in winter. But these harsh variables that are never even thought twice about in commercial gyms, made my journey something unique as it proved that no matter how uncomfortable the conditions are, you can still push through them and make progress. These difficulties and uncomfortable conditions sculpted the mind too and helped to increase my ability to step out of the comfort zone of training in temperate and 'nice' conditions, and enter the progress zone.

Below is the initial setup of the garage gym, when I first started buying equipment. A bench, barbell and a few dumbbells at first, gave me so much versatility to do new exercises, such as barbell bench press, dumbbell rows and pretty much any other free weight exercise that could be done in a professional gym. The floor space at the time was tiny, probably only taking up a bit more room as a super-king bed. Floor space does not matter, very few pieces of equipment requires very little room. However so much can be done with these very few pieces of apparatus as well as in very small spaces. The addition of an adjustable rack helped massively to allow me to perform squats and hold the barbell at different heights, but this is not necessary for beginning, as squats can be supplemented by doing dumbbell squats. No matter what the circumstance, there is always a way around them when it comes to training your body.

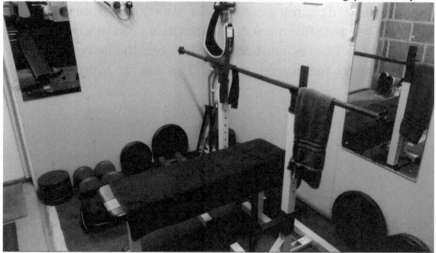

In this garage gym I made my first surge of muscle growth. My back grew from chin ups from the rafters and so did my chest from endless pushups and bench presses. Leg days were always interesting as the bench press rack did not have any safety catches to catch the barbell if I failed the squat -and sometimes it was much needed luxury. But I couldn't afford a huge power rack, nor did I have the space to store it, so I decided to use light weight and rep it out to compensate for its lightness.

One time I remember it was absolutely freezing, I had a little oil heater throbbing heat from the corner of the room and I had the squat bar loaded up really light with about 130 pounds on it. My leg days are never heavy as it is not safe to squat without a proper rack, so I relied on using high rep ranges to force the legs to grow. I un-racked the weight and squatted for ten reps. "easy! another ten, lets go!", I persisted to double my initial goal and reached twenty. "Again! another ten!", the cold made it so hard to breathe and this was becoming an endurance event as I had just reached thiry reps of squats. Now there was a vintage Bodybuilder from the 1980's, Tom Platz, who was made famous for the way he trained legs. He would squat for reps after reps after reps, with such heavy weight. Platz's training psychology was that there were "always five more" reps left in you, and that you have got to do whatever it takes to reach these last few reps that seemed impossible. I remember using this mindset and churning out another twenty reps from using this theory of reaching five more reps. Ultimately I had reached 50 reps! My legs shook from exhaustion. I couldn't breathe fast enough to compensate for the oxygen I needed. This was the byproduct of hard work and it definitely paid off when it came to getting stronger

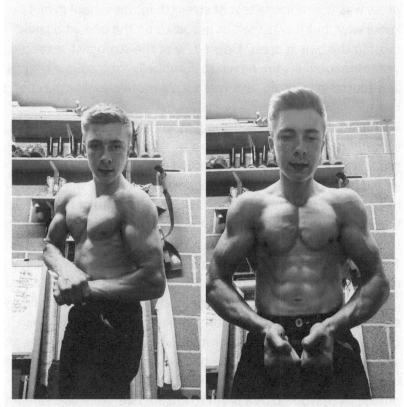

legs.

So after training in a cold and dark garage, I noticed that I had gained some pretty impressive lean muscle mass, for my age. And at that time I was only just old enough to join the school's gym. This excited me as this would be the first time I could train with the proper machines and equipment that I had witnessed all of the amazing bodybuilders like Dorian Yates using in the magazines and documentaries like Pumping Iron.

I can remember the first time entering the gym. There was a feeling of awe within me as I couldn't believe that finally I could use all of this high-tech equipment. My first session was chest, as it was my favourite to train. A Sixth-former, several years older than me, showed me how to properly bench press and we trained together for the next few weeks. After several months of constant training, there grew a small gang of us, my friends and a few older lads who would train together and spot each other. The dumbbell bench press was the ultimate test of strength in this school gym. I don't know why, but it was seen as heroic to be the one who could lift the most in the bench press. Only a few of the strongest seventeen-year olds could lift the heaviest Dumbbells for a couple of reps and as a fourteen year old, this was such a motivational aspiration to reach.

Within a few months I had completed half of the rack's weights, something of which was unheard of amongst the rest of my year group. Crowds of lads my age would gather around the bench as I would hoist these massive dumbbells up onto my thighs and lay back and press them. Looking back, it was a load of hype as I use them to warm up with now, but at that time, I was quite strong in that lift for my age and body weight.

Teachers were unhappy with this. They preached safe lifting with a minimum of twenty reps per set for every exercise. This forced everyone to lift light and in order to lift heavy we had devised a series of codes to communicate with each other to say when it was clear to roll out the heavy dumbbells from under the towles and attempt to lift them. A couple of times a few coaches would catch us and sit the group down to instill the dangers of lifting heavy, at our age. We worked as a team to ensure everyone was safe and were having fun but we also acted as catalysts to growing each other's ego. There were lads much taller than me and had more bulk, but I still could out-lift them, however this was becoming unhealthy when they became stronger as I was training to the redline of my limits to maintain this reputation.

Then when I was about fifteen I lifted the heaviest dumbbells for several reps of bench press. Nobody had bench pressed thirty kilos before in my year group, not for a select few in another two year groups ahead of mine, it was an accomplishment that everyone was proud of me for and this feeling was so motivating as hard work, my hard work, had finally paid off.

People became motivated by my lifts and would ask to train with me. It grew so busy that lads had to book a certain day to lift weights with me because I was already in high demand. I just loved helping people improve at their goals. I'd train with them and show them how to properly perform the exercises. I remember somebody wanted to train legs for one session with me, so I put them through their paces and they never returned the next week because they could not find the mind-set that was required to push through the pain barrier. Hard work means hard work and that's what it takes to build the best version of yourself. Everyone was moved with how intensely I trained and how it took it seriously. I wanted to try my best, so I trained my hardest and trained seriously.

When the GCSE exams came about, I had to leave this tradition behind and focus on my studies. I would say I only lifted weights once or twice a week, and that was at home in the garage gym. I did not train at the school facility any more after this. My physique did not drop too significantly as I managed to use the short training time, as maintenance work to preserve my muscles, but strength massively declined.

Then once the exams had finished, for my Sixteenth Birthday I enrolled at the commercial gym down the road from me. This gym was far better than the school gym, there were full sized barbells, a massive dumbbell rack with weights reaching fifty kilograms! From June to January I hit the gym hard. Most nights I would be in there pumping away, focusing on a different muscle group each session. During my time at the gym I noticed a surge in strength. My bench press was getting bigger and so was my deadlift. The deadlift quickly became my favorite lift as the feeling of lifting heavy weights stimulated so much impressiveness and accomplishment within me. In June time, I was struggling to pull about 135KG for a few reps. I wanted to reach 150KG before I went back to school in September. So I worked extremely hard at my deadlift and all the accessory work included to strengthen the back and the legs. By November, I was pulling 180KG for singles. This was incredible. Again, it was such a satisfying feeling to see myself break through a personal goal and achieve something difficult.

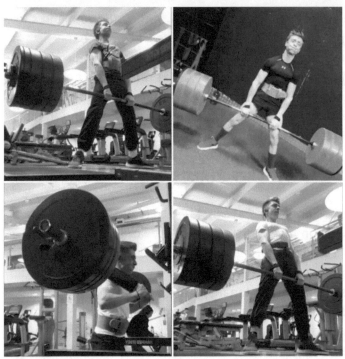

After Christmas, I had a friend that invited me to his Crossfit gym. This style of training was completely new to me and definitely challenged every muscle within me to keep up. After an hour of the grueling Crossfit workout of endurance work, we set up a barbell to work on deadlifts. I remember they had colourful Olympic plates which we messed around with to make a rainbow barbell.

In that gym, there was a feeling of community as everyone knew each other and spoke and chatted to nearly everyone they saw. So when they saw this new guy on their patch they were asking my mate who I was. "He's the deadlifter I was talking about. The one who does the Sumo!". And the guys would gasp as they'd hear this, as it is apparently a difficult variation of the lift. The sumo deadlift had become my method of deadlift, mostly because it worked well with my body-mechanics and how my hips worked and my long arms, despite being short.

We started off with about 70KG to warm up with. My mate tried the sumo but couldn't connect with it as it was so obscure to the conventional deadlift. It's an acquired taste I guess. We loaded the bar up though the 100KG mark. If I remember correctly he peaked at about 140 ish, my mate was a talented crossfitter whereas I professed in static lifts. The results of that session was:

150KG for 11 reps.

175KG for 5 reps.

180KG for 2 reps.

185KG for a single lift, making my new personal best.

Then I would attempt 190KG. I loaded the bar up, cranked-up the speakers in the gym and set myself into the zone. I strapped myself to the bar with my wrist straps and crouched at the bar for a good minute, preparing myself for the lift. My mate recorded the lift on my phone. The way I get into the mindset for a heavy lift is to reach the 'dark palace'. This nasty part of the mind that you go to to find anger or fear or something that will make all Hell-fire break loose when you commit to the lift. I reached a very vivid image within my mind, something that when I screwed my eyes up, I could see, plain as day.

I readied myself. Rolling the bar out in front of me, then rolled it back to my shins to commit to the pull. The bar slowly raised up. Above my knees. Then stopped just below lockout. I'd lost the potential of the driving force and couldn't muster any more power to finish the lift. Suddenly, I felt a twinge behind the leg. This shunted all the energy out of the lift, forcing me to drop the weight. As I dropped the barbell and stood up, the blood raced to my head, making me dizzy and so then I stumbled a few paces backwards before falling on my arse from the lactic acid and tightness in the leg. Luckily it was not a serious injury and I still continued to workout. Lifting heavy brought consequences with it. I was out of the gym for nearly two weeks as my back as well as my hamstring had been worn and worked to their limits. Therefore this was an important message to be learned and that you have to respect the exercises. Afterall we were in the gym for more than three hours straight lifting and pushing our bodies to their max, straight after having a few days off and indulging ourselves over Christmas.

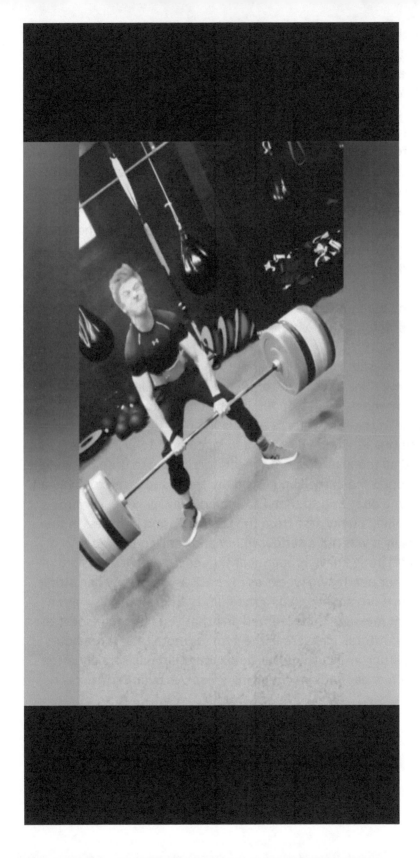

After recovering from the minor injury, I decided to stay clear from 90% max lifts and focus on refining my bodybuilding and becoming muscular rather than trying to hulk-up as much brute strength as possible. The body can only work at its maximum level for so long without needing a break. Professional Powerlifters cannot live the full year in peak condition as it will cause them injuries if they train their competition max lifts every session. I had learnt that this period of months was my lead up to my max lifts. They were a gradual progression of personal bests every other week as well as huge surges in the ability to perform heavy weights for reps. But then this was the aftermath of greatness, as I had not listened to the body and so I eventually turned down the weight to help keep healthy and continue training.

As January rolled into February, I was re-jigging my training styles, aiming to put on muscle mass whilst maintaining good strength on the side. This meant that I would concentrate on increasing my rep ranges as well as the overall volume and variation of exercises. To train to become as strong as possible in exercises such as the deadlift, you practice the one and only lift that will get you there: the deadlift. This is because the body has to become well practiced at what it will be doing, therefore apart from a few accessory squat and row work, nothing else will compliment your progression other than straight sets of just deadlifting. Whereas to build a killer physique, the body has to be trained in many different ways, variations and methods. Take for example you want to build a bigger and thicker back, you cannot just do pull-ups because the trapezius muscles and lower back muscles will be neglected and thus you will not have a complete back. To effectively train and sculpt a complete set of muscles, you need to train in different angles of attack. So this means that instead of just vertical pulling for the lats, you do horizontal pulling or rowing for the mid-back for thickness, then pulling upwards from the ground in the form of deadlifts and T-bar rows. Now the body, or back in this instance, is being targeted at multiple angles and will be fully worked to create as much muscle mass as possible. This can be applied to any other muscle group too, the more angles and variation of stress that can be placed upon them, the greater the results because they will have to adapt and ultimately grow larger to compensate for the resistance placed upon them.

In late March when the gyms closed due to the tragic CoronaVirus outbreak, I hit a brick wall. This would mean that training at home would be the only option to maintain my schedule. There was definitely enough weight equipment to keep me working out at home and plenty of weights to maintain my strength level. But I had become too comfortable training in a warm, bright and state of the art facility and that training at home would be like going back to the past without electricity. It would be a huge shock to the system. It was cold and dark and it required the mindset that I once had to be able to endure the coldness and the bland, brick walls. As the weather became nicer, I took the weights and bench outside and lifted there but I had just lost all motivation. School work, as well as a relationship I could not enjoy because of distance, havocked my headspace. I woke up, did my school work at my desk for hours, got back-ache and eye-strain from sitting at a screen. I'd be constantly texting my then-partner, with nothing new to talk about, adding to the monotony of the day. Then when I'd finish my work, I would have little to no motivation to workout. My dreams had been washed away by the ensnarement of lockdown and the loss of my happy place. The gym. The gym was the one place that I could improve and enjoy seeing my hard work pay off. Now I was working hard doing school work, but it was not the same, there was no variation of the day and it killed my dream of getting muscular and strong.

April, May, June, July, August, September, October and a chunk of November were all the same blur of repetitive dullness. Even when the gyms opened back up momentarily, I did not return. When schools opened for a bit and its social aspect, I still had lost all motivation and drive to become the best version of myself in the gym. However in late November I broke up with my then Girlfriend, and within a few hours, something had changed. I wasn't sad or depressed anymore. As horrible as it sounds, I didn't miss her or feel guilt and I quickly moved on without batting an eyelid. I was happy. My old pre-lockdown self was back. I could sleep better, I was laughing more. But most importantly I was able to sit down and think about my own journey, dreams and aspirations without the responsibility of looking after the happiness of others. I was free. Ultimately this gave me the power and thinking time to push on and progress with my career path, what car I wanted and most importantly at the time, the way I would get back into the gym. Or home gym.

Within days of the breakup, I was dusting off the dumbbells and cranking up the stereo to commence lifting again. My strength had been depleted to a shocking level. I was lacking the endurance to push when the training became tough. But this was not going to be the nail in the coffin of my bodybuilding journey. Weeks of progressively getting stronger brought me to my best physique yet. My power lifts were not as strong due to the minimal amount of weights I had but I remember lifting a 180KG deadlift as well as 100KG for twenty reps with a resistance band wrapped around to make it harder. I was back in the game, and so was my physique. I was hitting back and bicep shots in the mirror again, something that I had lost months ago to the lack of interest.

So January of the year 2021 was my comeback to the road of bodybuilding. The home gym became my happy place again, where I could dedicate an hour each night to brutally hard work as well as work on my mental focus and forge hardness and resistance to negativity within the mind.

That was my short story. Only the first few years of my life, but they were action-packed and filled with so many powerful and passionate dreams in which I invested every modicum of energy into, because I had a vision and a dream. These visions and aspirations made me rich because they made me happy> I started building a legacy in which I look back on and feel so proud of what I have achieved and done. My achievements might be warm-up numbers to what others can do and be washed away in belittlement like footprints in the sand. But they were my achievements and the memories and the people I met on this journey has sculpted a foundation of belief and confidence within myself.

Now it's your turn to fabricate big dreams with passion because when there is vision and enthusiasm, there will always be a way to excel in anything you put your mind to.

Ben Doughty

INTRODUCTION

Bodybuilding is not just a sport, it is an art. A Bodybuilder's mind is like a sculptor's, but instead of carving stone, they build muscle. As a sculptor he would use his different chisels for details and definition, instead of chisels, a Bodybuilder would have an inventory of exercises to develop one's muscle: size, proportion, clarity and symmetry. If an artist wants to develop a composition, they will add pencil and paint. Whereas a Bodybuilder exercises and uses different training methods to build the desired muscles, however it is harder and slower because they are making alterations on the human body.

Unlike other sports, Bodybuilding, like other weightlifting disciplines is a twenty-four hour lifestyle, in which you live bodybuilding, you eat, you train; you sleep bodybuilding, there is no secret formula, just hard work and dedication,motivation and concentration. Bodybuilding is a way of life. The building of mass and strength cannot be supplemented or divided into a team effort like in football or a relay team, in Bodybuilding, it is just you alone in the gym and an arsenal of exercises and principles to force the muscles to grow!

We all want the impressive physique of a superhero. That desire to resemble the figure of a Greek God and to have the strength of a grizzly bear. There's nothing more satisfying than having chiseled abs, a muscular chest and stunning leg muscles and the feeling of accomplishment and success after training hard. And in this book, I will teach you to train smart; ultimately gaining you faster results. For centuries muscularity has always been marveled throughout all cultures and the person who could carry the heaviest stone or who had the greatest physique would be crowned the strongest and a champion amongst the other competitors. This book is your instruction manual to begin the journey of becoming a champion. Sounds pretty good, doesn't it? This book will have the answers to the bookshelf of questions you will have about starting training. How can I get defined abs? How can I train at home with little or no equipment? What do I need to do to cut down fat? All in good time. This text will provide you with all the knowledge and encouragement to succeed and to progress along your own journey to gaining a superb physique, strength and overall fitness.

HOW DO MUSCLES GROW?

The human body is amazing! From a microscope's perspective, there are trillions upon trillions of tiny cells that are the foundation of tissue growth and repair and are a key feature in the development of the body. On a larger scale, there is the respiratory system which is responsible for the exchange of gases for the healthy intake of oxygen and the dispel of carbon dioxide, and then there is the nervous system which is the brain, spinal cord and complex system of nerves, in which control the response to external environments and how the body reacts to the stimuli. The more visible aspects of the body are the skeletal system: the framework of the body and the structure in which holds us upright. And finally, the muscular system, this series of tissues which collaborate to provide the bones with the power to move, and with the use of strength training they can become much more than the body's mechanism of movement. They can be trained for feats of strength and toned for aesthetics.

When you exercise, muscle fibres are broken down under the stress of the movement and load placed on the muscle. For example when performing a bicep curl, the two heads of the bicep: the long and short, will become forced to work to counter the weight and act in resistance to curl it. Their function is to act as a hinge (at the elbow) and contract the arm. As a result, the fibres of the biceps will tear and break-up, this is good damage! The damage caused by the lifting will be repaired by proteins and cell reproduction over a rest period, usually between 24-48 hours. In time, the bicep muscle along-side the nervous system will become more resistant against the stress of the movement and therefore will be able to tolerate it for longer; thus making the exercise easier.

Muscle Building Tip: GET AS MUCH BLOOD INTO THE MUSCLE AS POSSIBLE: One of the key objectives within a workout is to break down as many muscle fibres as possible, this is done through increasing the intensity or volume of the exercises to expose the muscles to more stress and resistance. Then it is important to fill the muscles with blood. This is called the pump and it is very satisfying as it increases the size and vascularity of the muscles temporarily; adding to a feel-good factor of having big muscles and satisfaction when posing in the mirror. Blood is full of oxygen and when there is lots of blood pumping around the body and filling the muscles, more nutrients can be injected into the muscles and will ultimately give them the energy needed to perform and will help with the replenishment of torn and damaged fibres with all the proteins and amino acids they require.

A way to describe this break-down and rebuilding of muscles could be seen as a brick wall being fixed after cracks appear. Builders, like proteins in the body, re-fill the gaps in the wall with cement , thus repairing the tears in the muscles and making them as good as new but slightly more resistant to stress.

Muscles over time become resistant to the same stress being placed on them, this means that they will not adapt and grow as they are capable of performing the same exercise without difficulty. In consequence, the muscles need to be 'shocked' with new principles, in which the body is not used to. This could be heavier weights in the style of progressive-overload, more repetitions or completely different exercises. The best way to ensure constant improvement in the muscles and strength, is to change up the routine and to add new challenges to make the muscles work more intensely.

EXERCISING FOR MUSCLE GROWTH

All exercise can be put into two general categories: Aerobic and Anaerobic. Both of these types of exercise are important for a well-rounded physique and level of fitness. Some sports will require either one or the other, but it is still important to incorporate them into all training programmes.

AEROBIC EXERCISE:

Aerobic exercise comes for the word 'aerobic' meaning 'with oxygen', and is the emphasis on the cardiovascular system and sustained periods of exercise that demands oxygen. Muscles need oxygen for respiration in order to function properly. As a result exercise such as running or swimming demands a constant supply of oxygen as it relies heavily on how efficiently the body can intake oxygen and distribute it to continue to power the muscles in use.

ANAEROBIC EXERCISE:

This form of training is a completely different set of principles to how Aerobic affects the body and what it is used for. Anaerobic means 'without oxygen' consequently forcing the body to make energy without the intake of oxygen during the exercise. These exercises are commonly performed at a higher intensity as the body cannot maintain power without oxygen to fuel its systems. Exercises such as the deadlift or events such as short distance sprinting or plyometric jumps, require a level of anaerobic ability due to their explosive nature. For example a 100 meter sprint is a test of absolute speed and how fast an athlete can run. The high speed often can only be maintained for this distance and cannot be sustained for much longer. Why? Because the body has such a high demand for energy to allow it to run fast, there is almost no way possible for the amount of oxygen or nutrients needed in such a large quantity over the period of time. Alongside this, many muscle building exercises and regimes rely on anaerobic power as they potentially last no more than 30 seconds such as a bench press or squat.

THE BENEFITS OF EXERCISE:

As well as getting in incredible shape, exercise has some other great benefits that are good for wellbeing and your health.

1. <u>Mental Health boost</u> : Exercise stimulates the brain to release endorphins. These chemicals are what makes the body feel good and as all animals do, we all strive to gain these feel good factors. Exercise can help to take your mind off your worries and you become focused on the present, this can really help you deal with a bad day from school or work as it helps clear the mind from the day. Running is one of the best after a stressful day because it is inexpensive, it can be done at any time of the day, you can decide where to go and it can be a good way to explore the area around you. Parks are a good running location as there's tranquil scenery and there's little traffic.

2. <u>It can grow your social time</u> : If you can exercise with a friend, it can boost social time and be a good time to laugh and enjoy company whilst getting in a good workout and it doesn't feel like work when you're laughing and talking to friends whilst you're lifting weights. Overall it's a good way to improve fitness as well as having fun. You might make new friends with similar fitness interests as you and you'll learn new training styles the more you workout with your training buddies.

3. <u>Organ Health</u> : Exercise can play a massive role in keeping the internal and important organs healthy and maintaining correct function. Predominantly aerobic exercise that taxes the lungs and circulatory system can have a significant positive effect on the effectiveness of the heart and lungs. The heart is a muscle and when worked to a standard of good fitness, it becomes more efficient at pumping blood around the body, ultimately needing less energy to function and making it easier to supply the body with oxygen. When somebody harnesses a good level of fitness there is a vast decrease in the likelihood of the onset of high blood pressure and heart disease, this is mainly due to the circulatory system being able to function without strain and doesn't have to work extra hard to keep the body regulating at its resting rate.

TRAINING FOR MUSCLE MASS

Now we have covered the basics of exercise and how the body works in response to exercise, we are now going to delve into the crystal-clear methods in which can be used to build muscle size and definition.

Firstly, to build lean muscle mass, the muscle needs to be worked under a degree of resistance, as this will force the breakdown of the muscle with micro-tears. Micro-tears are the foundational point of muscle growth as this is the initial 'damage' applied to the muscle. These micro-tears will then heal to form new muscle tissue which will be stronger and more resistant to strain and stress.

The resistance applied to muscles in weight training can be done by the following two exercise types.

ISOLATION EXERCISES:

These exercises focus on the use of a single joint to carry out a range of motion, consequently allowing singular muscle groups to be targeted. An example of this would be the dumbbell bicep curl. During this exercise, the elbow is the only joint in use, as it flexes the bicep as the weight is lifted. Only the bicep is worked here and is therefore isolated and has to perform the movement by itself without the recruitment of secondary muscle groups to help. As a result we can often see that isolation exercises such as leg extensions, bicep curls and shoulder lateral-raises cannot be done with heavy weight as the singular muscle has to work independently.

Isolation exercises are a good way to individually target lagging muscle groups. They can be good to even out a muscle imbalancement or to help strengthen a muscle after an injury. Due to the fact that these exercises restrict you from lifting heavy weights, it reduces their effectiveness to build a significant amount of mass. Secondly only one muscle is used here so secondary muscles are not activated, this too reduces the potential to build muscle mass as only a small percentage of the total body's muscles are being worked here.

However there is still a place in a workout for isolation exercises. When used correctly they can be powerful and be used to build intensity within a workout; securing maximal gains and muscle growth. Isolation exercise should be used in conjunction to Compound exercises (the next topic) as they will be used as the movements to finish the workout or to work specific areas and exhaust chosen muscle groups. For example, an athlete may be training their chest and focus their workout on the bench press-a compound lift. But may want to add extra emphasis on the pectoral muscles with the dumbbell fly. As a result of this, the athlete will further exhaust the chest without the use of secondary muscles, therefore solely intensifying the usage and direct targeting of the pectoral muscles.

COMPOUND EXERCISES:

On the contrary to isolation exercises, compound exercises rely on multiple joints and muscle groups to carry out a movement. The range of motion will require the targeted muscle to be worked (primary muscle) as well as several other muscles to help stabilise and complete the range of motion (secondary muscles) As a result of this vast muscle activation, more effort is needed and more muscle fibres are stressed. This increased scale of resistance will ultimately increase the amount of micro-tears across more muscle bodies, this means that once they have recovered, more of the muscular system will have been made stronger. An example of a compound movement is the barbell squat. Initially we think of the squat to predominantly work the thigh muscles. Breaking this down we can deduce that there are several muscles working together to secure the lift and range of motion. Firstly the quadriceps muscle (front of the upper leg) is activated, which is responsible for knee flexion and extension. Next the hamstring muscles (back of leg) are worked because they work in equilibrium with the quadriceps muscles to allow the contraction and bending of the leg. These two muscles alone are some of the largest in the body and together can move a considerably more amount of mass than a small bicep muscle in comparison, thus solidifying the effectiveness of the compound lift. In addition to these muscles, there are several more activated within the squat. The gluteus maximus (backside) is the body's most powerful muscle and allows for hip movement, this is important for a dynamic and full range of motion within any squatting movement. Then there are the abdominal muscles being worked to help stabilize the trunk and the erector spinae muscle in the lower back, keeping the body upright and preventing the body from collapsing or twisting when under the heavy weight.

As a result we can clearly see that these secondary muscles work as stabilisers within the squat and will adapt during recovery, and therefore will increase the overall development of the muscular system.

HYPERTROPHY AND MUSCLE BUILDING

Hypertrophy simply means the growth of muscle cells for greater muscle mass. Muscles grow under the influence of exercise, proper nutrition and recovery. It is important to understand that anaerobic exercise will allow the body to build lean muscle mass due to the fact that this style of training allows for the most effective way to breakdown of muscle fibres to eventually be repaired during recovery and thus multiply for muscle growth. The simple formula for muscular growth is to use the application of resistance to the exercise and in return, will tear the muscle fibres; forcing them to adapt and grow bigger and stronger.

The most effective exercises for absolute muscle growth are compound lifts. This is because more muscles and multiple joints are used, allowing more weight to be lifted, therefore creating more micro-tears within the muscle bellies. Comparing this to an isolation exercise, where only a limited amount of resistance can be used, compound lifts will allow you to target much more surface area of the body's muscular system with greater levels of resistance.

Hypertrophy requires a specific training style that differs from strength or endurance training. For training for absolute strength such as a Powerlifter, you would be training in the repetition range of between 1 to 5 reps. As this style of training requires maximal muscle activation and lasts for a very short, but extremely intense period of time. Then on the flip-side, endurance training for athletes such as Taekwondo fighters or Rowers, would train within the rep ranges of 20 plus reps. Sometimes even more, upto 50! Now for hypertrophy the standard rep range is suggested at between 8 and 15 reps. Some say: 8 to 12 and others say, 6 to 15. In all honesty, it all comes down to the individual person. Certain athletes respond well to high rep ranges and will experience the greatest muscle growth at around 12 to 15 reps whilst others might find that between 6 and 8 reps is perfect for their peak hypertrophy.

In summary, the muscles respond to changes in their day to day activity. When they are subjected to resistance, they grow stronger and larger to accommodate the work. So if a muscle is worked at 8 to 12 reps then it will become very good at training in that particular repetition range and in time, become used to this period of time under tension and adapt accordingly. However if the muscles are suddenly subjected to a completely new or different approach to training then their equilibrium is disrupted. So therefore they must adapt to gain capability to handle the new workload. This dramatic change in activity is called the 'Shocking principle', made famous by the great 7 time Mr Olympia, Arnold Schwarzenegger. This technique is where the athlete will change up their workout, weight, rest time and rep ranges to 'surprise' the muscles and to ultimately shock them into growth. Therefore when the rep range is changed after a period of time, then the muscles will be forced to adapt and in return grow.

STRENGTH TRAINING

Similar to hypertrophy, the body will become stronger when working against resistance. Instead of growing bigger, strength training will make the muscles stronger and more powerful to allow the body to work under greater loads. After a period of time when the body works against a heavy load, it will eventually become an easier task than it initially was. Why? Because the body adapts to external factors and stresses and becomes stronger. Strength training must be taken at a different training angle than hypertrophy training. This is because strength training relies on forcing the body to lift to its maximal capabilities in order to make the muscles stronger.

Commonly, strength training is harnessed by Powerlifters and Strongmen in which they rely on maximal muscular strength and the ability to lift extremely heavy weights. A Bodybuilder aims to shape the muscle and to build fullness, symmetry and an aesthetic balance throughout the entire body, as their goal is to attain the 'perfect physique'. On the flipside of this, Powerlifting and strength sports do not have their physique as a priority, or have the desire for chiseled abdominals or bulging biceps. Instead they purely focus on moving as much weight as possible and setting new personal records. So physique is not a priority.

The objective of lifting as much as possible has to be approached in a specific style of training: heavy weightlifting for short bursts of time. Usually Strength athletes will follow a programme that looks greatly different to a Bodybuilder's. This is because in order to improve maximal strength, they have to practice moving heavy weight to stimulate the body to react and become stronger. Unlike endurance athletes that can perform endless repetitions with light weight and have sets lasting for a couple of minutes, a Powerlifter or Strength athlete has to use much heavier weights so can only perform for a few seconds per set. This is why many Strongman programs have very few reps per set but have many more sets than endurance lifters or Bodybuilders. This is because volume is a key factor when it comes to any type of training. An endurance athlete may only need three sets of thirty reps per exercise, whereas a Powerlifter may need ten sets of only five reps to gain enough volume for the particular body part.

Strength athletes will perform exercises within the rep ranges of between 1 and 6 reps. Sometimes the objective is to lift a weight that is >95% of their one-rep max to force the body to make their maximum performance become a routine lift so the body gets used to intensive stress and thus has to adapt, consequently making the lift easier.

Compound lifts such as the: squat, bench press, deadlift and shoulder press are the foundation of all strength movements. These are the body's natural movements and have been used to test strength throughout history. Also, these movements are all compound lifts and are the exercises where the body is in the greatest position to move the highest amount of weight possible. These compound movements use large areas of secondary muscles and stabilisers therefore the muscles can become stronger in proportion to each other as the entire muscular system is recruited in exercises such as the deadlift and all work together as one unit for maximal efficiency.

POWERLIFTING

This discipline of training revolves around three competition movements: the squat, bench press and deadlift. A Powerlifter works to improve each of the three exercises to ultimately lift the heaviest weight possible in the exercise. In a Powerlifters competition or 'meet', the heaviest weight lifted of each of the three exercises is combined to form a 'total' and this is what the athletes are ranked on, based on their total lifts. Powerlifters use strength training principles to help improve their maximal strength for their three lifts. Every workout revolves around a particular lift, so variations of the lift will be carried out, as well as accessory work which gives the athlete different ways to improve their maximal effort in the main lift. For example, when training to improve the deadlift, an athlete may use rack-pulls to help improve the upper portion of the lift. This is where the bar is situated at a higher starting position than in a conventional deadlift, therefore making it easier to pull more weight. This variation will focus on the mid to end section of the deadlift and allow the athlete to work on the latissimus dorsi, trapezius and glute engagement. Other accessory exercises such as shrugs or grip exercises may be performed in training to develop lagging or weak points which will help to improve the athlete for when they come to compete with the conventional lift.

POWERBUILDING TRAINING

This style of training is when the idea of lifting heavy weight and becoming incredibly strong, is met with the technical training principles of Bodybuilding to allow an athlete to harness impressive strength whilst working on an aesthetic physique and keeping all muscle size proportionate with the symmetry and clarity as a physique athlete like a Bodybuilder would work towards.

Powerbuilding uses a combination of training principles from both Bodybuilding and Powerlifting. Compound lifts such as the squat, bench press and deadlift are the staple movements within nearly all Powerbuilding workout plans as they can be utilised for both strength building as well as hypertrophy. However, unlike Powerlifting, Powerbuilding harnesses a range of low rep ranges for power as well as high rep ranges for longer times under tension for the hypertrophy aspect of the program and this gives a broader scale of intensity variations and types of exercises. Isolation exercises that are used to target individual and specific muscles are used within Powerbuilding, more so than Powerlifting as they act as crucial movements to define the mass built by the heavy lifts to create the definition and detail required for bodybuilding.

Overall, Powerbuilding is an interesting style of training and can be both functional and fun as multiple training styles can be implemented. Furthermore, the workouts will be less monotonous because Powerbuilding requires the athlete to use different levels of intensity and therefore creating a wide spectrum of ways to build a workout, making lots of variation.

BODYBUILDING

Bodybuilding is the sport of developing the aesthetics of the entire body. The legs, back, chest, shoulders, arms and abs must be proportionate and symmetrical to each other. Originally bodybuilding was founded by the great Arnold Schwarnenegger who made the sport famous initially in the 1960-70s by bringing his physique to America and attaining 7 Mr Olympia titles. Ever since, Bodybuilding has become a growing sub-culture throughout the world and continues to become popular in every town and city gym.

This sport requires a level of discipline that is harder to foster than in other sports. Nutrition and eating clean and healthy meals, in large quantities, is a huge commitment which will determine a champion Bodybuilder to a novice. The training is intense too for competitive Bodybuilders too, every muscle group needs to be trained and some professionals train upto six days per week! Now in everyday life, hobbyist Bodybuilders do not need to meet the heavy requirements of eating like a horse and training several hours a day. But it is important to realise that this is a discipline that requires a very high level of consistency and hard work because anything that requires you to work the human body, albeit physio after an accident or Bodybuilding itself, constant work and commitment is required to improve and develop.

THE BODY IS LIKE GEOGRAPHY:

In higher level geography we learn that the world is one big system, made up of lots of smaller systems: feedback loops and all run at an equilibrium. Now the idea that the body is a system-like the world-means that we regulate at our own levels of equilibrium where homeostasis balances temperature within the body and changes how the body reacts to cope in different environments. In the world's systems it is clear that when its equilibrium is disrupted by an external force, it will eventually adapt and self-regulate to gain back normality. This is similar within the body as we too, have mechanisms to fight off disruptions whether that is infections in which our antibodies fight-off or damage inflicted on the body through exercise that when we recover, our muscles grow stronger to become more effective next time it is face to face with the same kind of resistance.

SHOULD YOUNG PEOPLE LIFT WEIGHTS?

This section focuses on the widely argued predicament concerning the effects on the growing teenage body from weightlifting. Firstly there has not been many studies done to prove the idea that teenagers should not lift weights, however there have been many arguments made that if it is done correctly for healthily improving muscular endurance and strength rather than trying to break records and go beyond their physical limit, at such a young age. In most gyms, there is an age restriction of sixteen or eighteen years and upwards. This is predominantly due to insurance and potential hazards which could occur within a gym and the maturity level of young people in such an environment.

Many young people (ages between 10 and 16) play or compete in some sort of physical sport, whether that being: football, track and field, netball, hockey; rugby. All of these activities will have a demand on the cardiovascular system and will tax their muscular endurance, as a result of this, the body is under the requirement to repair itself and to become stronger. Sports such as swimming and tennis, have a relatively low impact on the body and do not come with many potential risks to the athletes. These activities will require the athletes to exert a level of effort and will tax both the muscular and cardiovascular systems, resulting in 'soreness' the next day. Therefore this suggests that some level of strength training can be applied into the routines of younger people. The objective within a sport is to become either: faster, improve agility, improve coordination, grow stamina levels etc. So therefore this means that the body is forced to adapt to improve at the sport (in a gradual and healthy way) This idea means that we can deduce that lightweight or low-impact resistance training for increased muscular strength can be used by young teenagers if correctly supervised and carry out exercises under strict form regulations.

If a young person- for example a 13 year old- personally had the desire to begin to lift weights, then there is a safe and healthy way for them to carry out training. The important factor here is that 'they' must want to do it as weight training is a serious discipline and can be hazardous when concentration is not at its fullest. Whereas when a young person has the want to lift weights, then they will be more inclined to listen and carefully lift the weights in the correct manner. This links similarly to why young people are not permitted to enter a gymnasium before the ages of sixteen or eighteen years old.

Young people should ideally work with bodyweight exercises as the body should be capable of working with its own mass. Pushups, situps and running are good starting points in any workout programme and are great staple movements for young people when starting training. Bodyweight exercises can be done anywhere, they are inexpensive and can be done and learnt by virtually anyone and therefore creating a feel good factor because there is a feeling of achievement when you can accomplish a series of exercises.

In Bodybuilding, Powerlifting and endurance work, there are specific repetition ranges for specificity to ensure the athlete trains in the correct levels of intensity for their sport. This can be applied to resistance training for young people and fabricated in such a way to ensure both safe and fun lifting. higher repetitions with low weights is the ideal formula for any beginner lifter as well as youths, due to the fact that it gradually gets the muscles used to being placed and working under resistance. This low level of resistance will mirror the amount of resistance applied on their bodies to some of the sports they play. In sports such as track sprinting or swimming, the body is using muscle groups to power them across the field or through the water and has to withstand the mass of the individual whilst performing within the sport. This is relatively low resistance however activities such as running and jumping will have a level of impact on the body. This being said, the use of very light weight potentially will not create any more risk than what could be caused by the side-effects of running or jumping. Therefore to conclude this idea, young teenagers should be advised to work with light weight in the high rep ranges.

When working out, a young teen should be working in the repetition ranges of at least fifteen to twenty reps. This will prevent the onset of injury and will encourage the development of ligaments & tendons, as well as the healthy growth of bone density. This idea that the youth is lifting for higher repetitions is a safe way to encourage gradual improvements in muscular endurance as well as strength. However 'Weightlifting' should be avoided at this young age. Weightlifting is the discipline to train to lift weights in which are heavy and to beat records. This is the type of weightlifting seen in many gyms across the country as there is a competitive nature and a set of records to work towards. Training for maximal strength should be avoided by children and young teenagers because their bodies have not finished growing or fully developing, thus any injury could sustain permanent effects on their body.

We sometimes see child prodigies on the Internet who are impressively strong for their age or have a level of muscularity which is far beyond the orthodox standards of children of their age. These examples of extremely young people lifting weights or Bodybuilding are argued as being dangerous as well as some people saying it is perfectly fine. When we examine the average young teen, for example a thirteen year old, it is clear that they have not yet finished growing and are nowhere near as developed as a full grown adult. This means that lifting heavy weights could have an impact on their growth and development, and depending on the level of development the individual has, will give indication to their suitability to lift weights. As a result of this, some children who may have very rare or impressive genetics could have the potential to withstand greater amounts of resistance at a young age, have faster repair and recovery times and ultimately have a greater physical ability to withstand stresses on the body. This being said, any child or young teenager will have a physical limit to what they can lift or how much muscle they can build, this is due to hormone levels such as Testosterone. Testosterone begins to raise during puberty and is the 'Alpha Male' hormone. This hormone allows for the development of muscle as well as strength. So this clearly demonstrates that no matter how hard a child may train, there is a limit to how much muscle they can build and strengthen.

In conclusion to this endlessly debated subject, there is a clear line that should not be crossed when inspiring children to lift weights. Firstly the child or young teenager must want to lift weights and have a genuine level of enthusiasm that will allow them to be sensible and sustain concentration in order to remain safe whilst lifting. Secondly they must have a level of maturity too, as this will have a tremendous impact on their safety when performing exercises and in a training environment. Tertiarily, the young person must train within their comfortable level and must not exceed their level of training ability. As a result, they should either train with bodyweight exercises only or compound movements such as bench press, squats, shoulder press and deadlifts, if carried out under the supervision of a responsible adult. They must perform these exercises correctly and with strict form. Lastly, the athlete must train within a high repetition range with very light weight in order to allow them to stimulate the muscles enough for results, whilst limiting the risk of injury or strain.

THE EXERCISES

Now that you have a basic understanding about how the body reacts to training and the different types of training goals, it is time to learn the exercises and how they can be used to build impressive strength and sculpt lean muscle mass.

THE SQUAT

Squats are the bread and butter movement for leg and lower body development. Why? Because they recruit the largest muscles of the body, making them stronger and more powerful, as well as allowing you to burn the most amount of calories due intensive usage of energy and multiple muscle groups taxed within this exercise. Just to name the main muscles worked here include; The Quadriceps, Hamstrings, Glutes and calves. These are some of the largest muscle bellies within the body and help contribute to overall power and strength when performing other exercises as well as in sports. Other muscle groups such as the lower back and abdominals will be placed under resistance in order to keep the body straight and aligned, therefore the squat will help shred belly-fat and build a strong back.

The amazing thing about squats that make them so easy to perform is that they can be done with just bodyweight alone as well as their brilliant compatibility with dumbbells and barbells. In truth, the barbell squat will build the most muscle mass as it forces the body to work (squat) under a heavy load, and in return will grow stronger. Despite this, bodyweight squats and dumbbell squats are still greatly effective as they can be performed with high reps as well as with individual legs for advanced exercise, in order to maximise their effectiveness when they become easier.

To Perform the squat, stand tall with a straight back and your feet placed slightly wider than shoulder-width apart. With your back in a neutral position, squat down to a comfortable level, making sure that you keep your abdominals braced and chest up. When you are as low as you can comfortably go, or when your knees are bent at a right angle, push through your heals and explode upwards to complete the movement. Remember to keep your back straight and keep a controlled movement.

For the barbell squat, position the barbell on a sturdy rack at shoulder or trapezius height. Next position yourself underneath the barbell with your shoulder-blades pinched back and rest the bar onto them. This will help to keep the bar in a safe and rigid position. Next carryout the squat, ensuring that you do not go too low beyond a 90 degree bend in the knees, or this could cause knee issues. Gradually lower into the squat with your chest facing up to help keep the spine in a comfortable position as well as helping you keep balanced. Especially with the barbell squat, remember to keep the back straight and abs braced, to prevent any injury. From the lowered position, use your legs to drive the barbell upwards to the first position.

When standing with the barbell on your back, never lock your knees,as this can put too much stress on the joint, remember to keep a slight bend in the knee as this will distribute the load and keep your joints healthy.

As this is a compound exercise, the squat should be a huge staple within the leg workout. For beginners, aim to include 3 to 4 sets of 12 reps of weighted squats into your workout. However if you do not have any equipment, aim to carry out as many reps as possible for 3 sets. Rep ranges above 20 will help burn unwanted fat and will also help aerobically and develop your cardiovascular system.

THE BENCH PRESS

The bench press is the king of all chest exercises. It is one of the most well known and easiest exercises to perform to develop a strong set of pectoral muscles.

Like the squat, the bench press can be done with both a barbell and dumbbells, therefore making it very versatile and adaptable with limitations of space and equipment. Unfortunately it cannot be done with bodyweight however the pushup is a very reliable alternative to help pack on great muscle and improve muscle definition, without the need of any equipment at all.

When I first started weight training, I could not afford a bench press so I would use the floor as this allowed me to practice a very similar range of movement of the bench press. Corners of sturdy coffee tables and the corners of beds can be used to allow you to replicate the clearance on either side of the body for the arms to lower in order to gain a better stretch.

However the bench press is most effective with a standard bench that can be bought relatively cheaply for about £50/ $50.

Lay down on the bench, with the barbell secured on the rack just under an arms reach away. Pinch your shoulder-blades back when setting up as this will help with mobility and deltoid health. Keep the back flat on the bench with your feet planted on the floor at either side. Balance is formed with your base so it is vital to have a solid set up before you begin to lift. Once your foundation is ready, unrack the barbell with your hands placed at shoulder width on the bar. A narrow grip will target the triceps more as a secondary muscle and help with arm development, whereas a wider grip will focus on gaining a great stretch on the pecs and help to build a wide chest. Once you have decided on your grip, lower the bar slowly, with your elbows tucked in close to your body. If the elbows are flared out to the side, this can cause damage to the shoulders and make the lift uncomfortable. Likewise in any exercise, only use a weight that you can perform safely and with good form. Lower the bar until it is almost touching your sternum or chest bone, then push the bar in a straight line up towards the ceiling. Use the chest and triceps to drive the bar. Like the squat, never lock-out your arms or this will place stress on the elbow, so try to keep a slight crease in the elbow when the exercise is being performed.

When Performing the bench press with dumbbells, you will be using a very similar technique, however the movement of the dumbbells from the floor to your ready position is important to get right. Sit on a bench with your chosen dumbbells on either side on you. Pick them up and place them on your knees, when you have an even grip on the weights, use the knees momentum to push the weights up as you roll back onto your back. This technique can be difficult at first but practice with light dumbbells will quickly help hone in your ability to work with heavier weight. Once laying on the bench with the dumbbells above you, lower them to chest level and after a pause at this position, raise them up back to the beginning position. After you have completed your set, carefully sit up with the dumbbells and use your knees to safely transport them as you get to a seated position.

Bench pressing is one of the key exercises to maximise chest development, therefore it should always be used within an upper body session. On an adjustable bench, the bench press can be performed at an incline as well as a decline position. These set-ups will help target different portions of the chest such as the upper head and mid chest. All the above principles apply to the incline and decline variation, however always be sure to use a weight that you can lift comfortably when trying new exercises.

BENT-OVER ROW

Many beginner lifters neglect the back muscles purely because you cannot see them and they are much harder to connect with mentally because of this barrier when training. Whereas with chest training, you can see the pectorals contract and stretch under the resistance as well as you can 'show-off' the chest as everytime you look into the mirror you want to see improvements, and many of us never have the desire to train muscles that we cannot see, such as the back and calves and the majority of the posterior chain.

The bent over row can massively help to boost your muscularity of the back as well as secondarily work the biceps. The middle section of the back will be predominantly worked here however the lower back as well as as high as the trapezius muscles will be worked to a great extent too.

This exercise can be performed with both dumbbells and with a barbell, and the technique is very much identical with both.

First set up a barbell or pair of dumbbells with a weight that you can comfortably lift for 12 to 15 repetitions. Have the bar in front of you and stand with your feet facing forward and in a shoulder-width stance. For the barbell row, bend down with a straight back and grasp the bar with an overhand grip. Your grip should be wider than your stance so ultimately your hands are on the outside of your knees. From this lowered position, keep a neutral spine and push through the heels to pick the bar up to hip level. Now you should stand up straight with your chest up and shoulders pulled back: as if you are standing to attention at a military parade. With this set up, try to lower your position to as close to parallel with the floors as possible. This will help to engage the back during the lift. Once you are in a comfortable bent-over position, pull the barbell towards your abdominals and squeeze the upper back while rowing the barbell towards you. Remember to keep a straight back and do not arch as this will cause injury. As you lift heavier weights, invest in a weightlifters belt as this will help to brace the core and back to ensure a healthy alignment of the back when lifting.

These same principles can be applied to the dumbbell row, instead of holding a barbell, you carry out the exact same procedure as before but with two independent weights on either side of your body.

SHOULDER PRESS

The shoulder press is an amazing compound exercise in which allows you to work the bulk of the shoulders as well as target the triceps muscles too. The shoulder is composed of three heads: the Anterior (front), Medial (side), and the Posterior (rear). All three heads of the deltoid will help you deliver the effect of a three dimensional shoulder as well as attain freakish strength in the upper body.

Begin with a barbel loaded with your desired weight, we will be aiming to reach 12 to 15 reps as a beginner. Like in the bent-over row, set your foundation with a shoulder-width stance and proceed to lift the barbell to hip height. Always keep a solid and neutral back when lifting any piece of equipment. Next you will carry out what is known as a 'clean'. This means to throw the barbell up to shoulder level in a controlled and safe manner. With the barbel at hip height, bend at the knees and drive upwards, this will give you enough leverage to pull the barbell up to collar-bone height and set you up into the beginning of the shoulder press.

The exact same method should be used for dumbbell presses too for shoulders.

Next you will push the barbell up over-head and pause at the top of the repetition. Remember not to fully extend your elbows as this will place unnecessary stress on the elbow joint. Once you have pressed the weight above your head, gradually lower the bar back to collar-bone height and go for another rep.

This exercise can be done with so many different implements, and can be done with such little equipment too. Sandbags and buckets can be used to press with as well as any other stable object that is heavy enough to be manipulated and pressed over-head.

THE BICEP CURL

This exercise is probably one of the most well-known weightlifting exercises. The bicep curl, as the name implies, is an isolation exercise in which allows you to concentrate on targeting the bicep. Bicep curls are a very simple yet effective exercise to perform as well as being very easy to do without lots of equipment.

First stand with two dumbbells at your sides which are loaded at a comfortable weight which are not too heavy to use. Next you must keep your elbows locked-in by your sides and curl the weight up. This movement should look like you are closing a hinge. Your arm begins straight down by your sides and as you curl the weight, you hinge at the elbow and contract the bicep. Once the dumbbell is at its highest point of the curl, pause and squeeze the bicep. This is important because it will force as much blood into the muscle and blood carries the nutrients needed to fuel muscle growth. Then slowly lower the dumbbells down back to your sides, whilst continuing to keep your elbows tucked in close to your sides.

Bicep curls can also be done with a barbell and is a mirrored technique to dumbbell curls, however the bar will restrict your range of movement within the wrists, so this may be uncomfortable for those with tight joints or joint issues.

THE DEADLIFT

The deadlift is considered to be the most 'Alpha' and impressive lifts within the gym. It consists of you picking up a loaded barbell to your hips and controlling the bar back down to the ground. The athlete to perform the heaviest deadlift is heavily praised to be the strongest of people due to the intensive recruitment of nearly all of the body's muscles. This exercise requires the usage of the back, hamstrings, glutes, trapezius a well as the shoulders, arms and calves. The deadlift is the ultimate compound lift to build the most impressive level of strength. However the deadlift is one of the most dangerous exercises if performed incorrectly therefore it must be respected and done carefully and properly.

First load the barbell with a light weight, as you should not be going heavy when practicing the deadlift technique. Set your feet up behind the bar in a shoulder to hip-width position as everyone's biomechanics and limb length will slightly differ and change individual preferences to how wide their feet are. Once you have found your comfortable footing position, plant your feet solidly into the floor.

Next bend at the hip, squatting down with your chest up and back aligned. Grasp the bar at shoulders width and ensure that you are centered in the bar to certify good balance. Your grip should be with your hands in an 'over-hand' position, you can use the 'over-under' set up which consists of one palm facing up and the other facing downwards when holding the bar. The double-over hand is the safest as it will ensure better stability and reduce the risk of bicep tearing.

At the bottom position of the lift where you are squatted down, push through your feet and legs and drive the bar upwards. The aim is to stand up with the barbell and contract the glutes to finish the movement. When you are standing up from the squat, remember to keep everything rigid and tight. Keep the back and core braced and straight as any curvature or arching will oppose a danger to back and spinal health. Use light weights at the beginning because this will help you gain a feeling for the lift whilst practicing the technique.

IMPORTANT EXERCISE HABITS

When you exercise it is extremely important to prepare the body for the intensity it is about to endure. Therefore the warmup is a critical process to go through as this will protect the body from injury as well as help increase the mobility of the body for the upcoming session. A similar process must be carried-out at the end of every workout, called the cool down as this will help to lower the heart rate and gently relax the muscles from a high intensity environment back to a resting state. As a result, the cooling down process prevents the body from injuring itself once a workout is finished. If an athlete has finished an intensive 1500M run, they will have a heavy build-up of lactic acid as well as a very high heart-rate. The cool-down will be a series of gentle exercises to help lower the pulse very slowly as well as help to flush away the toxicity within the muscles, such as lactic acid. The process of respiration includes the out-let of byproducts and this is important as it helps the body recover from the interval of intensity. If the body did not go through the cool-down process, the muscles could begin to cramp and recover at a much slower rate, therefore injuries are more likely to be made when training muscles that have not fully recovered yet.

WARMING UP

This initial stage of a workout is important because it helps to prepare the body gradually for the workout to come. Think of the body like a car engine, it would be dangerous to thrash a cold engine with high revs as the oil has not fully circulated around the engine and damages may be made. Likewise, the body must be warmed up and readied in order to commence a healthy and risk-reduced workout.

There are two main phases of a basic warm-up:
The pulse raiser and then sports specific stretches and movements.

First it is a good idea to go for a run or use a piece of cardio machinery. Running, rowing or cycling are a good way to increase the heart rate and can be used at all levels of experience. About ten minutes is a good time frame to aim for here as it will give the body time to pump oxygenated blood around the body as well as lubricate the joints with synovial fluid which will help with mobility and ease of movement.

Next you should practice movements that are specific to the sport or activity you are about to participate in. For example a runner will perform a series of lunges and short sprints or walking hurdles to help prepare the leg muscles and joints for the main running event. This practice will help mobilize the specific muscle groups for the workout or spot and prevent the onset of injury later on. It is important to keep specific to your activity or sport as there is very little point of warming up the biceps if you are doing a leg workout, because it should be the legs that are the primary focus of the mobility and warm-up process.

After your cardio and dynamic movements to warm-up the joints and muscles, static stretches are to be used to target specific muscles and stretch them. Stretching helps to get the muscles ready for the exercises and prevents knots from developing. Again it is important to keep sports-specific here as if you are training your chest, it is important to stretch the chest, shoulders and triceps muscles because they are the main muscles being worked here.

THE COOL DOWN

This process is equally as important as the warm-up as it is the process of gradually letting the intensity decrease. A sudden stop of intense exercise on the body can be dangerous, this is because the body needs to be gradually guided into recovery. The body uses a much higher heart rate to supply itself with enough oxygen when under aerobic and anaerobic stress, than when it is resting and requiring a constant and steady pulse. As a result of this, the heart rate must be lowered back to a resting level to allow the body to carefully go back into 'rest mode'. Furthermore cooling down includes stretches, similar to the warm-up. These stretches will open up the muscles and help to flush the unwanted lactic acid out of them and into the bloodstream. These waste products in the bloodstream will be respired out of the body.

The cool-down should begin with a light cardio session, this should be a low-resistance level of jogging, or cycling or rowing. This will gradually lower the heart rate and get the body used to the slowing of blood-flow and decreased speed of breathing. Next it is important to have a slow walk or cycle to further lower the heart-rate, this should take approximately 5 minutes and get gradually slower as time goes on. Once the heart-rate is at a much lower level, begin stretching the muscles you have been using in the workout. Concentrate on stretching individual muscles and holding the tension for 10 to 15 seconds before releasing and changing stretch. Hold the stretch for longer if you feel a particular tightness that needs to be addressed more thoroughly. Stretching should be done for roughly 5 minutes as this will give plenty of time to work through all of the muscles that have been used within the workout.

NUTRITION

Nutrition is the foundation of where all muscle and fitness gain take place. Without fuel, a race car will not be able to be powered on and win races. The body is similar, if there is not enough good macronutrients going into the body, it will under-perform and not provide you with enough energy to work at your best potential. The basic components of nutrition for muscle growth revolve around Carbohydrates, Proteins and Fats.

CARBOHYDRATES

Carbohydrates are the building blocks of energy and are the main principle for fueling the body and providing it with enough energy to stay functioning throughout the day. Carbs are made up of different chains of starches and sugars found in food which can be broken down and burnt to make the body's energy. Foods such as rice, pasta, bread and potato are packed full of carbohydrates and are very important foods to give you plenty of energy for working out.

PROTEINS

This strand of macronutrients is the most composition for muscle growth. In short, proteins act as the recovery agents to allow muscles to grow and repair themselves. Proteins are a must when it comes to bodybuilding and weight training because the body is under constant need to recover and the process of protein-synthesis is very important to keep the muscles in their best condition. Overall, without protein you would not grow or have developed into the person you are today. Proteins build the living tissues of the human body and allow the growth of hair, bones, muscles and brain function. Foods such as eggs, red meat, dairy and soy beans are a huge contributors to a protein-rich diet as they have such a high continent of good quality proteins.

FATS

Many people think that the concept of fat is nasty and should be avoided. However there is a split between good and bad fats. Bad fats can be deduced as saturated fats in which are hard to break down and do not compliment a healthy lifestyle. Saturated fats can be the root cause of many diseases such as heart disease, stroke and high cholesterol levels. Foods such as pizza, sweets and other fast food and processed foods contain a high saturated fats content and must be consumed in moderation to maintain the practice of healthy-eating.

On the other hand, good fats such as unsaturated fats are essential to keeping a healthy body. Omega-3 is an important fat that is found within foods such as salmon. These series of fats are crucial for aiding healthy brain and eye function as well as helping heart function. As a result foods with good fats should not be avoided as they can contain the nutrients needed to help with the healthy function of tissues and organs. Foods such as nuts, avocados and fish are a great source of healthy fats that heal and mend the body.

PROTEIN SUPPLEMENTS

In many gym environments, there is a large hype about taking whey protein and creatine powders to aid performance. However these supplements are not as critical to your gains to what is said in the media and by fellow gym members. A supplement is basically a formula of synthetic ingredients in which you usually mix with water to create a drink. This drink will contain a rich concentration of proteins, amino-acids as well as electrolytes and other nutritional elements. However many people rely on these protein drinks alone, to make improvements to their game. The clue is in the name of these powders: 'supplement'. To supplement means to use something different instead of your usual product, in order to accomplish something. In this case, a protein supplement is used to take the place of a meal. When you do not have the time to eat a proper meal, you will have a deficit of calories and nutrition, therefore a protein shake will provide you with a fast installment of all the essential macronutrients that the body needs.

Protein supplements should not be relied upon as the source of all nutrition. Instead, your daily meals should be the primary focus of gaining all the essential carbohydrates and proteins needed for the day. The usage of the protein shake should be an addition to the amount of meals you have per day. For example, if you have 5 meals per day as an amaeture bodybuilder, you would fit your protein drink on top of that. The same goes for someone who eats 3 meals per day, meals should never be replaced by protein powders, complemented with them.

The best time to consume a protein drink would be after you have finished a workout. There is a period called the anabolic window straight after a workout, where whatever food you eat in that time frame, will get used in the immediate processes of muscle recovery. Therefore the recommended intake of protein shakes are best consumed straight after a workout is complete.

Personally I have never used a protein powder. Many lifters around me have fallen for the trap of the enchanting drink and have still been outlifted by the 'natural' yours truly. My point is that protein drinks are only necessary if you cannot consume enough natural foods to fuel your workouts. Natural food has the greatest and best quality proteins and are as pure and healthy as nutrients get. Protein shakes are made in factories and out of synthetic products, therefore you are ingesting a product that is not technically natural or healthy in the long run.

The misuse of supplements can lead to health concerns and really hinder the organ quality. Take the kidneys for example, they flush out impurities and clean the many litres of blood within the body. If the body is now full of impure and chemically produced products, then they will have to work harder and ultimately strain.

In conclusion, protein powders do not make an athlete any better than the next. They will not give you 20 inch biceps or a 500 pound squat, but they can be used to aid in the intake of essential nutrients in which the body needs for repair and function.

CLOSING MESSAGE

Now I hope that after reading this book you have learnt something. You may be a complete beginner to bodybuilding and have now been able to understand the concepts of muscle building and kick-start your journey. Or you may already have been training for a few years and now have an extended knowledge about essential training methods. Wherever you stand in the experience scale, you should all take away the same teaching. Motivation. Motivation is the only element you will ever need to excel at something. Reading about healthy eating might just be enough to fuel your own beginning to cut out saturated fats in order to improve your diet. Or maybe reading my short story may have helped you understand that you don't really need much equipment to start lifting weights, but by having a dream, you can use every piece of energy to make the best of what you have, to fuel your journey to where you want to be.

Just remember that everyone starts somewhere and that you cannot reach your goal without going the distance to get there.

Made in United States
Troutdale, OR
11/20/2023

14767033R00030